# Low purine Diet

Nutritional guide for beginners

**Bailey J. Heath**

# Contents

# Chapter One

# PURINE LEVEL IS LOW.

## PURINE LEVEL IS LOW.

A low-purine diet restricts high-purine foods. Purines are a type of naturally occurring substance that can be found in a variety of foods. Purines aren't necessarily harmful, but excessive amounts should be avoided. Purine is broken down by the body into uric acid, which is a waste product. Uric acid crystals forming in the joints can lead to a variety of health problems. Kidney stones and gout, a form of arthritis, are two of the most common.

A low-purine diet isn't meant to completely eliminate purines. Rather, the goal is to keep track of how much purine you're taking in. The foods and drinks to avoid and limit are listed below. Learning how your body reacts to purine-containing foods is beneficial.

## 1. Honey-Roasted Cherry and Ricotta Tartine

35 minutes total Ingredients/Servings: 4

• 1 tablespoon honey, plus more for serving • 1 teaspoon lemon zest • 1 tablespoon lemon juice • 2 teaspoons extra-virgin olive oil • salt

1 cup part-skim ricotta cheese • 1 teaspoon fresh thyme • 14 cup slivered almonds, to taste Directions

Preheat the oven to 400 degrees Fahrenheit (200 degrees Celsius). Wrap parchment paper around a rimmed baking sheet.

2. Combine the cherries, honey, lemon juice, oil, and salt in a bowl and toss well. Roast the cherries in the prepared pan for 15 minutes, shaking it once or twice during cooking.

3. Make a toast. Ricotta, lemon zest, roasted cherries, thyme, almonds, and sea salt are sprinkled on top. If desired, add a drizzle of honey.

## 2. Sun-dried Tomato Cream Sauce with Chicken Cutlets

20-Minute Preparation 20 minutes total Ingredients/Servings: 4

12 cup slivered oil-packed sun-dried tomatoes, plus 1 tablespoon oil from the jar • 12 cup finely chopped shallots

2 tablespoons chopped fresh parsley • 12 cup heavy cream Directions

1. Season chicken with 1/8 teaspoon salt and 1/8 teaspoon pepper. In a large skillet over medium heat, heat sun-dried tomato oil. Cook, turning once, until the chicken is golden brown and an instant-read thermometer registers 165°F.

A thermometer inserted into the thickest part reads 165 degrees Fahrenheit after about 6 minutes. Place a plate on top of it.

2. Toss in the shallots and sun-dried tomatoes in the pan. 1 minute of stirring Raise the temperature to high and pour in the wine. Cook for about 2 minutes, scraping up any browned bits as needed. Reduce heat to medium-low and stir in cream, any remaining chicken juices, and the remaining 1/8 teaspoon salt and pepper; cook for 2 minutes.

Return the chicken to the pan and toss it in the sauce to coat it. Serve with the sauce and parsley on top of the chicken.

## 3. Potatoes in Melt

25 minutes to prepare 1 hour and 10 minutes (total)

Ingredients/Servings: 6

• 2 pounds Yukon Gold potatoes, peeled and cut into 1-inch slices • 2 tablespoons melted butter • 2 tablespoons extra-virgin olive oil • 2 teaspoons chopped fresh thyme • 1 teaspoon chopped fresh rosemary • 34 teaspoon salt • 12 teaspoon ground pepper • 1 cup low-sodium vegetable broth or chicken broth Directions

1. Preheat oven to 500 degrees F. Place rack in upper third of oven.

In a large mixing bowl, combine the potatoes, butter, oil, thyme, rosemary, salt, and pepper. In a 9-by-13-inch metal baking pan, arrange the cookies in one layer. (Avoid using a glass dish because it may break.) Cook for about 30 minutes, flipping once, until browned.

3. Carefully pour the broth into the pan, along with the garlic cloves. Continue roasting for another 15 minutes or until the broth has mostly evaporated and the potatoes are very tender. Warm it up and serve.

## 4. Cauliflower Casserole with Cheesy Ground Beef

30 Minutes Preparation 30 minutes total
Ingredients/Servings: 6

1 pound lean ground beef • 3 cups bite-size cauliflower florets • 3 garlic cloves, minced • 2 tablespoons chili powder • 2 teaspoons ground cumin • 1 teaspoon dried oregano • 12 teaspoon salt • 14 teaspoon ground chipotle • 1 (15 ounce) can no-salt-added petite-diced tomatoes • 2 cups shredded extra-sharp Cheddar cheese

Directions

1. Preheat the oven to 350°F and place the rack in the upper third. Increase the temperature of the broiler to high.

2. In a large oven-safe skillet, heat the oil on medium. Cook, stirring occasionally, for 5 minutes, or until onion and bell pepper have softened. Cook, stirring and breaking up the beef into smaller pieces, for 5 to 7 minutes, until it is no

longer pink. Cook for 1 minute, stirring in the garlic, chili powder, cumin, oregano, salt, and chipotle. Bring the tomatoes and their juices to a simmer, then cook, stirring occasionally, for another 3 minutes, or until the liquid has been reduced and the cauliflower is tender. Turn off the burner.

3. Top with sliced jalapeos and cheese. 2 to 3 minutes under the broiler, or until the cheese is melted and browned in spots

Preparation Time: 40 minutes 5. Spicy Weight-Loss Cabbage Soup 1 hour total Ingredients (servings): 8

• 2 tablespoons extra-virgin olive oil • 2 cups chopped onions • 1 cup chopped carrot • 1 cup chopped celery • 1 cup chopped poblano or green bell pepper • 4 large garlic cloves, minced • 8 cups sliced cabbage • 1 tablespoon tomato paste • 1 tablespoon minced chipotle chiles in adobo sauce • 1 teaspoon ground cumin • 12 teaspoon ground coriander

• 2 (15 ounce) cans rinsed low-sodium pinto or black beans • 34 teaspoon salt • 12 cup chopped fresh cilantro, plus more for serving

• For garnish, crumbled queso fresco, plain nonfat Greek yogurt, and/or diced avocado

Directions

In a large soup pot (8 quart or larger), heat the oil over medium heat. Cook, stirring frequently, for 10 to 12 minutes, until onions, carrots, celery, poblano (or bell pepper) and garlic have softened. Cook, stirring occasionally, for another 10 minutes, or until cabbage has softened slightly. Cook, stirring, for 1 minute longer with the tomato paste, chipotle, cumin, and coriander.

2. Combine the broth, water, beans, and seasonings in a large mixing bowl. Over high heat, cover and bring to a boil. Reduce the heat to low and cook, partially covered, for about 10 minutes, or until the vegetables are tender. Take the pan off the heat and add the

lime juice, cilantro, and If desired, top with additional cheese, yogurt, and/or avocado.

6. 20-Minute Slow-Cooker Chicken & Chickpea Soup

4 hrs 20 mins total time

Ingredients/Servings: 6

• 12 cup soaked dried chickpeas • 4 cup water • 1 large yellow onion, finely chopped

4 teaspoons ground cumin • 4 teaspoons paprika • 14 teaspoon cayenne pepper • 14 teaspoon ground pepper • 2 pounds bone-in chicken thighs, skin removed, trimmed

14 cup halved pitted oil-cured olives • 12 teaspoon salt • 14 cup chopped fresh parsley or cilantro • 1 (14 ounce) can artichoke hearts, drained and quartered Directions

1. In a 6-quart or larger slow cooker, drain chickpeas. Stir together 4 cups water, onion, tomatoes with juice, tomato paste, garlic, bay leaf, cumin, paprika, cayenne, and ground pepper. Chicken should be added.

2. Cook for 8 hours on low or 4 hours on high, covered.

3. Remove the chicken from the pan and place it on a clean cutting board to cool slightly. Bay leaf should be thrown out. In the slow cooker, combine the artichokes, olives, and salt. Remove and discard the bones from the chicken before shredding. In a large mixing bowl, combine the soup,

chicken, and salt and pepper. Serve topped with parsley (or cilantro) (or cilantro).

7. Chicken & Spinach Skillet Pasta with Lemon & Parmesan

25 minutes to prepare Total Time: 25 mins
Ingredients/Servings: 4

• 8 ounces gluten-free penne pasta or whole-wheat penne pasta\s• 2 tablespoons extra-virgin olive oil\s• 1 pound boneless, skinless chicken breast or thighs, trimmed, if necessary, and cut into bite- size pieces\s• ½ teaspoon salt\s• ¼ teaspoon ground pepper\s• 4 cloves garlic, minced\s• ½ cup dry white wine

• Juice and zest of 1 lemon\s• 10 cups chopped fresh spinach\s• 4 tablespoons grated Parmesan cheese, divided

Directions

1. Cook pasta according to package directions. Drain and set aside.

2. Meanwhile, heat oil in a large high-sided skillet over medium-high heat. Add chicken, salt and pepper; cook, stirring occasionally, until just cooked through, 5 to 7

minutes. Add garlic and cook, stirring, until fragrant, about 1 minute. Stir in wine, lemon juice and zest; bring to a simmer.

3. Remove from heat. Stir in spinach and the cooked pasta. Cover and let stand until the spinach is just wilted. Divide among 4 plates and top each serving with 1 tablespoon Parmesan.

8. Lemon-Garlic Vinaigrette\sPrep Time: 5 mins Total Time: 5 mins Servings: 10 Ingredients

• ¾ cup extra-virgin olive oil\s• 5 tablespoons red-wine vinegar\s• 3 tablespoons lemon juice\s• 1 ½ tablespoons Dijon mustard\s• 1 clove garlic, grated\s• ¾ teaspoon salt\s• Ground pepper to taste Directions

1. Combine oil, vinegar, lemon juice, mustard, garlic, salt and pepper in a jar with a tight-fitting lid. Shake until well blended.

9. Slow-Cooker White Bean, Spinach & Sausage Stew

30 Minutes Preparation

Total Time: 15 hrs 50 mins

Ingredients/Servings: 6

• 2 cups dried cannellini beans\s• 5 cups unsalted chicken stock\s• 1 plum tomato, stem end trimmed (about 5 ounces)\s• 1 teaspoon kosher salt\s• ½ teaspoon black pepper\s• 4 garlic cloves, lightly crushed\s• 2 fresh rosemary sprigs\s• 6 ounces spinach-and-feta chicken-and-turkey sausage (such as Applegate Organics), cut diagonally into 1/2-inch-thick slices\s• 5 ounces baby spinach, roughly chopped\s• ¼ cup chopped fresh flat-leaf parsley\s• 2 tablespoons extra-virgin olive oil

Directions

1. Sort and wash the beans; place in a large Dutch oven. Cover with water to 2 inches above the beans; cover and let stand 8 hours. Drain the beans. Place the beans in a 5- to 6-quart slow cooker. Add the stock, tomato, salt, pepper, garlic, and rosemary sprigs. Cover and cook on LOW until the beans are tender, about 7 hours.

2. Lightly mash the bean mixture with a potato masher, breaking up the tomato and garlic. Add the sausage to the slow cooker; cover and cook on LOW until thoroughly heated, about 20 minutes. Add the spinach and parsley, stirring just until the spinach begins to wilt. Discard the rosemary sprigs.

Ladle the stew into bowls; drizzle evenly with the oil before serving.


## 10. Cabbage Roll Casserole

Prep Time: 35 mins 1 hour total Ingredients (servings): 8

• 3 tablespoons extra-virgin olive oil, divided\s• 1 pound lean ground beef\s• 1 cup chopped onion\s• 3 cloves garlic, minced\s• 2 cups low-sodium chicken or beef broth\s• 1 (15 ounce) can no-salt-added tomato sauce\s• 1 cup long-grain white rice\s• ½ teaspoon salt, divided\s• ½ teaspoon ground pepper, divided\s• 8 cups chopped green cabbage (1 1/4 pounds)\s• 2 teaspoons dried dill\s• ¼ teaspoon crushed red pepper\s• 1 ½ cups shredded Cheddar cheese

Directions

1. Preheat oven to 350°F. Lightly coat a 9-by-13- inch baking dish with cooking spray.


2. Heat 1 tablespoon oil in a large saucepan over medium heat. Add ground beef and onion; cook, stirring, until the beef is no longer pink, about 5 minutes. Add garlic and cook until fragrant, about 1 minute. Stir in broth, tomato sauce, rice, 1/4 teaspoon salt and 1/4 teaspoon pepper; bring to a

simmer. Cover, reduce heat to maintain a simmer and cook, stirring once or twice, until the rice is tender, about 17 minutes (the mixture will be a little saucy). Uncover and remove from heat.

3. Meanwhile, heat the remaining 2 tablespoons oil in a large skillet over medium heat. Add cabbage, dill, crushed red pepper and the remaining 1/4 teaspoon each salt and pepper. Cook, stirring, until the cabbage is just tender, 5 to 7 minutes. Turn off the burner.

4. Spread half the cabbage in the bottom of the prepared baking dish. Top with half the beef mixture then half the cheese. Repeat with the

remaining cabbage, beef mixture and cheese. Bake until hot and the cheese has melted and started to brown, about 25 minutes.

11. One-Pan Chicken & Asparagus Bake Prep Time: 15 mins 35 minutes total Ingredients/Servings: 4

• 2 (8 ounce) boneless, skinless chicken breasts, cut in half crosswise • 12 ounces baby Yukon Gold potatoes, halved lengthwise • 8 ounces carrots, diagonally sliced into 1-inch pieces • 3 tablespoons extra-virgin olive oil, divided • 2 teaspoons ground coriander, divided • ¾ teaspoon salt, divided • ½ teaspoon ground pepper, divided • 2 tablespoons lemon juice • 2 tablespoons chopped shallot • 1 tablespoon whole-grain Dijon mustard • 2 teaspoons honey • 1 pound fresh asparagus, trimmed

• 2 tablespoons chopped fresh flat-leaf parsley • 1 tablespoon chopped fresh dill • Lemon wedges Directions

1. Preheat oven to 375 degrees F. Place chicken on a clean work surface and cover with plastic wrap. Using a meat mallet, pound the chicken pieces to an even 1/2-inch thickness. Arrange on one half of a large rimmed baking sheet. Arrange potatoes and carrots in a single layer on the other half of the pan. Drizzle the chicken and vegetables with 1 tablespoon oil; sprinkle with 1 teaspoon coriander, 1/2 teaspoon salt and 1/4 teaspoon pepper. Bake for 15 minutes.

2. Meanwhile, whisk lemon juice, shallot, mustard, honey and the remaining 2 tablespoons oil, 1 teaspoon coriander, 1/4 teaspoon salt and 1/4 teaspoon pepper in a small bowl.

3. Remove the pan from the oven; switch the oven to broil. Stir the potato-carrot mixture; arrange asparagus in the center of the pan. Spoon the lemon juice-shallot mixture evenly over the

chicken and vegetables. Broil until the chicken and vegetables are lightly browned, asparagus is tender-crisp and a thermometer inserted in the thickest portion of the chicken registers 165 degrees F, about 10 minutes. Remove from oven; sprinkle evenly with parsley and dill. Serve with lemon wedges.

## 12. Loaded Broccoli Casserole

20-Minute Preparation Total Time: 55 mins Ingredients (servings): 8

• 3 slices bacon • 1 ½ pounds broccoli crowns, cut into bite-size florets • ½ teaspoon ground pepper • ¼ teaspoon salt • 1 tablespoon extra-virgin olive oil (if needed) • 1 ½ cups shredded extra-sharp Cheddar cheese, divided

• .666 cup reduced-fat sour cream • 4 scallions, sliced, divided Directions

1. Preheat oven to 425°F. Lightly coat a 9-by-13-inch baking dish with cooking spray.

2. Place bacon in a large nonstick skillet over medium heat; cook until crisp, 6 to 8 minutes.

Transfer to a paper-towel-lined plate to cool, then chop (reserve drippings in the pan).

3. Add broccoli, pepper and salt to the pan and toss with the bacon drippings until coated. If your bacon didn't render much fat, add up to 1 tablespoon oil; toss to coat. Transfer to the baking dish and roast, stirring once or twice, until tender, about 30 minutes.

4. Meanwhile, combine 1 cup cheese, sour cream and half the scallions in a small bowl. When the broccoli is tender, add the cheese mixture to the baking pan and stir to coat well. Sprinkle with the remaining 1/2 cup cheese and the reserved bacon. Bake the cheese is melted, about 5 minutes. Sprinkle with the remaining scallions.

## 13. Chicken, Quinoa & Sweet Potato Casserole

Prep Time: 15 mins Total Time: 45 mins Ingredients (servings): 8

• 4 cups cubed peeled sweet potatoes (about 1 pound) • 3 tablespoons water • 1 tablespoon canola oil • 1 ½ pounds boneless, skinless chicken thighs, trimmed • 2 cups chopped seeded poblano chiles • ½ cup thinly sliced shallots • 2 tablespoons minced garlic • 2 cups unsalted chicken broth • 1 ½ cups multicolored quinoa • ⅓ cup dry white wine

• 1 teaspoon kosher salt • 1 teaspoon ground cumin • ½ teaspoon ground cinnamon

• ⅛ teaspoon cayenne pepper • ½ cup crumbled queso fresco • ¼ cup fresh cilantro Directions

Preheat the oven to 400 degrees Fahrenheit (200 degrees Celsius).

2. Place sweet potatoes and water in a microwave- safe bowl. Cover with plastic wrap; pierce a few holes in the top with a fork. Microwave on High for 4 minutes.

3. Meanwhile, heat oil in a large skillet over medium-high heat. Add chicken and cook until browned, 4 to 5 minutes per side. Transfer the chicken to a clean cutting board and let stand 5 minutes. Cut into 1-inch strips.

4. Add poblanos, shallots and garlic to the pan and cook over medium-high, stirring occasionally, until the shallots are lightly browned, about 2 minutes. Add broth, quinoa, wine, salt, cumin, cinnamon and cayenne. Bring to a boil. Remove from heat and stir in the sweet potatoes and chicken.

5. Spoon the mixture into a 7-by-11-inch (or similar- size) broiler-proof baking dish. Cover with foil. Bake for 20 minutes.

6. Remove from oven; increase oven temperature to broil. Uncover the casserole and sprinkle with cheese. Broil 8 inches from the heat source until golden brown, about 5 minutes. Sprinkle with cilantro. Let cool for 5 minutes before serving.

## 14. Vegetable Weight-Loss Soup

Prep Time: 45 mins 1 hour total Ingredients (servings): 8

• 2 tablespoons extra-virgin olive oil • 1 medium onion, chopped • 2 medium carrots, chopped • 2 stalks celery, chopped • 12 ounces fresh green beans, cut into 1/2-inch pieces • 2 cloves garlic, minced • 8 cups no-salt-added chicken broth or low- sodium vegetable broth • 2 (15 ounce) cans low-sodium cannellini or other white beans, rinsed • 4 cups chopped kale • 2 medium zucchini, chopped • 4 Roma tomatoes, seeded and chopped • 2 teaspoons red-wine vinegar

• ¾ teaspoon salt • ½ teaspoon ground pepper • 8 teaspoons prepared pesto Directions

1. Heat oil in a large pot over medium-high heat. Add onion, carrot, celery, green beans and garlic. Cook, stirring frequently, until the vegetables begin to soften, about 10 minutes. Add broth and bring to a boil. Reduce heat to a simmer and cook, stirring occasionally, until the vegetables are soft, about 10 minutes more.

2. Add white beans, kale, zucchini, tomatoes, vinegar, salt and pepper. Increase heat to return to a simmer; cook until the zucchini and kale have softened, about 10 minutes. Top each serving of soup with 1 teaspoon pesto.

## 15. Melting Cabbage

20-Minute Preparation 1 hour total Ingredients (servings): 8

• 1 head green cabbage (about 2 pounds), outermost leaves removed • 4 tablespoons extra-virgin olive oil, divided • ¾ teaspoon salt, divided • ¾ teaspoon ground pepper, divided • 1 medium onion, halved and sliced • 4 large cloves garlic, sliced • 1 teaspoon caraway seeds • 1 teaspoon cumin seeds • 3 tablespoons tomato paste • 2 cups low-sodium chicken or vegetable broth • 1 teaspoon dry mustard • Chopped parsley for garnish • Whole-grain mustard for serving

Directions

1. Preheat oven to 350°F.

2. Slice cabbage in half through the root. Cut each half into 4 wedges, keeping the root intact. Heat 1 tablespoon oil in a large cast-iron or other heavy ovenproof skillet over medium heat. Add 4 cabbage wedges and cook until browned in spots on both sides, 3 to 5 minutes per side. Transfer to a plate and sprinkle both sides with 1/4 teaspoon each salt and pepper. Repeat with 1 tablespoon oil, the remaining cabbage and 1/4 teaspoon each salt and pepper.

3. Add the remaining 2 tablespoons oil, onion, garlic, caraway seeds and cumin seeds to the pan; cook, stirring, until starting to soften and brown, 2 to 3 minutes. Add tomato paste and cook, stirring, until starting to darken, about 2 minutes. Add broth, dry mustard and the remaining 1/4 teaspoon each salt and pepper; increase heat to medium-high and bring to a boil. Return the cabbage to the pan, overlapping the wedges if necessary. Bake, turning once, until the cabbage is

very soft and the sauce has reduced and thickened, 40 to 45 minutes. Sprinkle with parsley and serve with mustard, if desired.

16. Cabbage Diet Soup Prep Time: 35 mins Total Time: 55 mins Ingredients/Servings: 6

• 2 tablespoons extra-virgin olive oil • 1 medium onion, chopped • 2 medium carrots, chopped • 2 stalks celery, chopped • 1 medium red bell pepper, chopped • 2 cloves garlic, minced • 1 ½ teaspoons Italian seasoning • ½ teaspoon ground pepper • ¼ teaspoon salt • 8 cups low-sodium vegetable broth • 1 medium head green cabbage, halved and sliced • 1 large tomato, chopped • 2 teaspoons white-wine vinegar

Directions

1. Heat oil in a large pot over medium heat. Add onion, carrots and celery. Cook, stirring, until the vegetables begin to soften, 6 to 8 minutes. Add bell pepper, garlic, Italian seasoning, pepper and salt and cook, stirring, for 2 minutes.

2. Add broth, cabbage and tomato; increase the heat to medium-high and bring to a boil. Reduce heat to maintain a simmer, partially cover and cook until all the vegetables are tender, 15 to 20 minutes more. Remove from heat and stir in vinegar.

17. Sheet-Pan Salmon with Sweet Potatoes & Broccoli

30 Minutes Preparation Total Time: 45 mins
Ingredients/Servings: 4

• 3 tablespoons low-fat mayonnaise • 1 teaspoon chili powder

• 2 medium sweet potatoes, peeled and cut into 1- inch cubes • 4 teaspoons olive oil, divided • ½ teaspoon salt, divided • ¼ teaspoon ground pepper, divided

• 4 cups broccoli florets (8 oz.; 1 medium crown) • 1 ¼ pounds salmon fillet, cut into 4 portions • 2 limes, 1 zested and juiced, 1 cut into wedges for serving • ¼ cup crumbled feta or cotija cheese • ½ cup chopped fresh cilantro

Directions

1. Preheat oven to 425 degrees F. Line a large rimmed baking sheet with foil and coat with cooking spray.

2. Combine mayonnaise and chili powder in a small bowl. Set aside.

3. Toss sweet potatoes with 2 tsp. oil, 1/4 tsp. salt, and 1/8 tsp. pepper in a medium bowl. Spread on the prepared baking sheet. Roast for 15 minutes.

4. Meanwhile, toss broccoli with the remaining 2 tsp. oil, 1/4 tsp. salt, and 1/8 tsp. pepper in the same bowl. Remove the baking sheet from oven. Stir the sweet potatoes and move them to the sides of the pan. Arrange salmon in the center of the pan and spread the broccoli on either side, among the sweet potatoes. Spread 2 Tbsp. of the mayonnaise mixture over the salmon. Bake until the sweet potatoes are tender and the salmon flakes easily with a fork, about 15 minutes.

5. Meanwhile, add lime zest and lime juice to the remaining 1 Tbsp. mayonnaise; mix well.

6. Divide the salmon among 4 plates and top with cheese and cilantro. Divide the sweet potatoes and broccoli among the plates and drizzle with the lime-mayonnaise sauce. Serve with lime wedges and any remaining sauce.

## 18. Eggplant Parmesan

25 minutes to prepare Total Time: 45 mins
Ingredients/Servings: 6

• Canola or olive oil cooking spray • 2 large eggs • 2 tablespoons water • 1 cup panko breadcrumbs • ¾ cup grated Parmesan cheese, divided • 1 teaspoon Italian seasoning • 2 medium eggplants (about 2 pounds total), cut crosswise into ¼-inch-thick slices • ½ teaspoon salt • ½ teaspoon ground pepper • 1 (24 ounce) jar no-salt-added tomato sauce

• ¼ cup fresh basil leaves, torn, plus more for serving • 2 cloves garlic, grated • ½ teaspoon crushed red pepper

• 1 cup shredded part-skim mozzarella cheese, divided
Directions

1. Position racks in middle and lower thirds of oven; preheat to 400°F. Coat 2 baking sheets and a 9- by-13-inch baking dish with cooking spray.

2. Whisk eggs and water in a shallow bowl. Mix breadcrumbs, 1/4 cup Parmesan and Italian seasoning in another shallow dish. Dip eggplant in the egg mixture, then coat with the breadcrumb mixture, gently pressing to adhere.

3. Arrange the eggplant in a single layer on the prepared baking sheets. Generously spray both sides of the eggplant with cooking spray. Bake, flipping the eggplant and switching the pans between racks halfway, until the eggplant is tender and lightly browned, about 30 minutes. Season with salt and pepper.

4. Meanwhile, mix tomato sauce, basil, garlic and crushed red pepper in a medium bowl.

5. Spread about 1/2 cup of the sauce in the prepared baking dish. Arrange half the eggplant slices over

the sauce. Spoon 1 cup sauce over the eggplant and sprinkle with 1/4 cup Parmesan and 1/2 cup mozzarella. Top with the remaining eggplant, sauce and cheese.

6. Bake until the sauce is bubbling and the top is golden, 20 to 30 minutes. Let cool for 5 minutes. Sprinkle with more basil before serving, if desired.

## 19. Loaded Cauliflower Casserole

Prep Tim: 20 mins 1 hour total Ingredients (servings): 8

• 3 slices bacon • 1 head cauliflower (about 2 pounds), cut into bite- size pieces • ½ teaspoon ground pepper • ¼ teaspoon salt • 1 ¼ cups shredded sharp Cheddar cheese, divided • ⅔ cup sour cream • 4 scallions, sliced, divided Directions

1. Preheat oven to 425 degrees F.

2. Place bacon in a large nonstick skillet over medium heat; cook until crisp, 6 to 8 minutes. Transfer to a paper-towel-lined plate and let cool. (Reserve the drippings in the pan.)

# Chapter Two

## Recipes

3. Combine cauliflower, pepper, salt and the bacon drippings in a 9-by-13-inch baking dish. Roast, stirring twice, until tender, about 35 minutes.

4. Meanwhile, combine 1 cup cheese, sour cream and half the scallions in a small bowl. When the cauliflower is tender, stir the cheese mixture into the cauliflower in the pan. Sprinkle with the remaining 1/4 cup cheese. Bake until hot, 5 to 7 minutes more.

5. Chop the cooled bacon. Sprinkle the hot casserole with thebacon and the remaining scallions.

20. Sautéed Brussels Sprouts with Bacon & Onions

35 minutes total Servings: 10 Ingredients

• 2 ½ pounds Brussels sprouts, trimmed • 4 slices bacon, cut into 1-inch pieces • 1 tablespoon extra-virgin olive oil • 1 large onion, diced • 4 sprigs thyme or savory, plus 2 teaspoons leaves, divided • 1 teaspoon salt • Freshly ground pepper to taste • 2 teaspoons lemon juice (optional) Directions

1. Bring a large pot of water to a boil. If sprouts are very small, cut in half; otherwise cut into quarters. Cook the sprouts until barely tender, 3 to 5 minutes. Drain.

2. Meanwhile, cook bacon in a large heavy skillet over medium heat, stirring, until brown but not

crisp, 3 to 6 minutes. Remove with a slotted spoon to drain on a paper towel. Pour out all but about 1 tablespoon bacon fat from the pan.

3. Add oil to the pan and heat over medium heat. Add onion and cook, stirring often, until soft but not browned, reducing the heat if necessary, about 4 minutes. Stir in thyme (or savory) sprigs, salt and pepper. Increase heat to medium-high, add the Brussels sprouts, and cook, tossing or stirring occasionally, until tender and warmed through, about 3

minutes. Remove the herb sprigs. Add the bacon, thyme (or savory) leaves and lemon juice, if using, and toss.

21. Cauliflower Rice and Spinach & Artichoke Casserole

20-Minute Preparation 45 minutes total Ingredients/Servings: 4

1 tablespoon extra-virgin olive oil • 1 pound boneless, skinless chicken breasts, cut into 1-inch pieces • 14 teaspoon salt • 14 teaspoon ground pepper • 2 garlic cloves, minced • 1 (14 ounce) can quartered artichoke hearts, drained and chopped • 12 cup unsalted chicken broth • 4 cups cauliflower rice • 3 cups coarsely chopped fresh spinach

• 1 cup part-skim mozzarella cheese, shredded

Directions

Preheat the oven to 375 degrees Fahrenheit (190 degrees Celsius). Using cooking spray, lightly coat a 9-by-13-inch baking dish.

2. In a large pot, heat the oil on medium. Cook, stirring occasionally, until the chicken is opaque on all sides, about 4 minutes. Cook for 1 minute while stirring. Cook, stirring

constantly, for 3 to 4 minutes, until the liquid has reduced and the chicken is cooked through. Remove the pan from the heat and stir in the cauliflower rice, spinach, yogurt, and 1/2 cup mozzarella cheese.

3. Spoon the remaining 1/2 cup mozzarella over the top of the mixture in the prepared baking dish. Cook for 20 to 25 minutes, or until the cheese is melted and browning in spots. Before serving, set aside for at least 5 minutes.

Preparation Time: 30 Minutes 22. Chicken and Zucchini Casserole 1 hour and 25 minutes total

Ingredients (servings): 8

• 3 tablespoons butter, divided • 2 pounds boneless, skinless chicken breast, cut into 1-inch pieces • 2 large zucchini, cut into 1/2-inch pieces • 1 large red bell pepper, chopped • 13 cup all-purpose flour • 1 cup no-salt-added chicken broth • 1 cup whole milk • 3 ounces reduced-fat cream cheese • 14 cups shredded part-skim mozzarella cheese, divided

Directions

Preheat the oven to 400 degrees Fahrenheit (200 degrees Celsius). In a large skillet on medium-high heat, melt 1 tablespoon butter. Cook, stirring occasionally, for about 8 minutes, until the chicken is well browned. In a medium bowl, place the chicken. Cook, stirring occasionally, until the zucchini and bell pepper begin to soften, about 4 minutes. In the same bowl as the chicken, add the zucchini mixture.

2. Remove the pan from the heat and add the remaining 2 tablespoons of butter. Cook, stirring constantly, for about 1 minute or until the flour begins to brown. Bring the broth and milk to a boil while constantly whisking. Remove from heat and stir in 3/4 cup mozzarella and cream cheese until thoroughly combined. Add the pepper and salt and stir to combine. Remove the liquid from the chicken and vegetable mixture and stir it into the cheese sauce. Fill a 2-quart baking dish halfway with water and set aside. Sprinkle the remaining 1/2 cup of cheese over the casserole and place it on a foil-lined baking sheet.

3. Bake for 20 to 25 minutes, or until top is browned and edges are bubbling. Before serving, set aside for 10 minutes.

Prep Time: 35 minutes for 23. Parmesan Mushroom Casserole 1 hour total Ingredients/Servings: 6

• 14 cup extra-virgin olive oil plus 1 tablespoon, divided • 1 cup chopped onion • 3 garlic cloves, minced • 2 pounds baby bella mushrooms, sliced • 3 tablespoons all-purpose flour • 34 teaspoon salt • 12 teaspoon ground pepper • 12 cup sour cream

Directions

Preheat the oven to 350 degrees Fahrenheit (180 degrees Celsius). Using cooking spray, spray an 8-inch-square baking dish.

2. In a large skillet, heat 1/4 cup oil on medium. Cook, stirring occasionally, for 3 minutes, or until onion is soft and beginning to brown. Cook for 1 minute while stirring. Add mushrooms in batches, stirring and cooking them down a little before adding another handful, until they've lost their opaqueness but there's still some liquid in the pan. Cook, stirring constantly, for 1 to 2 minutes, until the vegetables have thickened. Remove from the heat and stir in the sour cream, 1/4 cup Parmesan cheese, 1/4 cup parsley, and the lemon juice. Place in the baking dish that has been prepared.

3. In a small mixing bowl, combine panko, the remaining 1 tablespoon oil, Parmesan, and parsley; toss to combine. Over the mushroom mixture, sprinkle the topping evenly. Cook for 20 to 25 minutes, or until the sauce has thickened and the breadcrumbs have lightly browned.

Dressing with lemon and scallions, no. 24

5 minutes to prepare 5 minutes in total Ingredients/Servings: 6

• 6 tbsp extra-virgin olive oil • 3 tbsp lemon juice • 2 tbsp chopped shallot • 1 tbsp honey • 12 tbsp salt • 14 tbsp ground pepper

1. In a small mixing bowl, combine the olive oil, lemon juice, shallot, honey, salt, and pepper.

25. Parmesan-Crusted Lentil and Vegetable Soup

15-Minute Preparation 40 minutes total Ingredients/Servings: 6

• 2 tablespoons extra-virgin olive oil • 3 cups fresh or frozen chopped onion, carrot, and celery mix • 4 garlic cloves, chopped • 4 cups low-sodium vegetable or chicken broth • 12 cup green or brown lentils • 1 (15-ounce) can unsalted diced tomatoes, undrained • 2 teaspoons finely chopped fresh thyme • 12 teaspoon salt • 12 teaspoon ground pepper • 12 teaspoon crushed red pepper

• Chopped fresh flat-leaf parsley for garnish • 12 tablespoons red-wine vinegar Directions

2. In a Dutch oven or a large pot, heat the oil on medium. Cook, stirring occasionally, for 6 to 10 minutes, until onion, carrot, and celery mixture is softened. Cook, stirring frequently, for 30 seconds, until garlic is fragrant.

3. Add the broth, lentils, tomatoes, thyme, salt, pepper, crushed red pepper, and, if using, Parmesan rind. On medium-high heat, bring to a boil. Reduce to medium-low heat; cover and cook, stirring occasionally, for 15 to 25 minutes, or until lentils are almost tender, adding water as needed to thin to desired consistency.

4. Add kale to the mix. Cook for 5 to 10 minutes, covered, until kale is tender. If you're using Parmesan rind, remove it and throw it away. Vinegar should be added now. Split the money in half.

Mediterranean Diet in a Slow Cooker (#26) 15-Minute Stew Prep

6 hours and 45 minutes total

Ingredients/Servings: 6

• 2 (14 ounce) cans no-salt-added fire-roasted diced tomatoes
• 3 cups low-sodium vegetable broth • 1 cup coarsely
chopped onion • 34 cup chopped carrot • 4 garlic cloves,
minced • 1 teaspoon dried oregano • 34 teaspoon salt • 12
teaspoon crushed red pepper • 14 teaspoon ground pepper •
1 (15 ounce) can no-salt-added chickpeas, rinsed, divided

• 3 tbsp extra-virgin olive oil • 6 lemon wedges • 3 tbsp extra-
virgin olive oil (Optional) Directions

In a 4-quart slow cooker, mix together the tomatoes, broth,
onion, carrot, garlic, oregano, salt, crushed red pepper, and
pepper. Cook for 6 hours on low, covered.

2. In a small bowl, pour 1/4 cup of the slow cooker's cooking
liquid. 2 tablespoons chickpeas, mashed until smooth with a
fork

3. Toss the remaining whole chickpeas into the slow cooker
with the mashed chickpeas, kale, and lemon juice. To
combine everything, whisk it together. Cook, covered, on Low
for about 30 minutes, or until the kale is tender.

4. Divide the stew among 6 bowls and drizzle with olive oil.
Basil leaves can be added as a finishing touch. If you'd like,
garnish with lemon wedges.

Chhole is number 27. (Chickpea Curry)

15 minutes total Ingredients/Servings: 6

• 6 tablespoons canola oil or grapeseed oil • 2 teaspoons ground coriander • 2 teaspoons ground cumin • 12 teaspoon ground turmeric • 2 14 cups no-salt-added canned diced tomatoes with their juice (from a 28-ounce can) • 34 teaspoon kosher salt • 2 15-ounce cans chickpeas, rinsed

• For garnish, fresh cilantro

Directions

1. In a food processor, finely mince the serrano, garlic, and ginger. Re-pulse after scraping down the sides. Pulse the onion until it's finely chopped but not watery.

2. In a large saucepan, heat the oil on medium-high. Cook, stirring occasionally, for 3 to 5 minutes, or until the onion mixture has softened. Cook, stirring constantly, for 2 minutes with coriander, cumin, and turmeric.

3. Pulse the tomatoes until they are finely chopped in a food processor. Salt and add to the pan. Cook, stirring occasionally, for 4 minutes at a low simmer. Reduce heat to a

low heat, add the chickpeas and garam masala, cover, and cook for 5 minutes more, stirring occasionally. If desired, garnish with chopped cilantro.

## 28. Casserole de Petits Fours de Noel de Noel de Noel

20-Minute Preparation 1 hour and 10 minutes (total)

Ingredients (servings): 8

• 14 cup chopped sun-dried tomatoes • 1 tablespoon extra-virgin olive oil • 2 garlic cloves, finely chopped • 12 teaspoon crushed red pepper • 1 teaspoon lemon zest • 2 cups low-fat milk • 5 large eggs • 1 cup crumbled feta cheese • 12 ounces rustic whole-wheat bread, torn into 1-inch pieces (about 8 cups)

Directions

1. Place the spinach in a clean kitchen towel and wring out as much liquid as possible over the sink. In a medium mixing bowl, combine the spinach and artichoke hearts.

2. In a small skillet over low heat, cook the tomatoes, oil, garlic, crushed red pepper, and lemon zest, stirring

frequently, until fragrant and golden brown, 3 to 4 minutes. Add the spinach mixture to it and mix well.

3. Preheat the oven to 350 degrees Fahrenheit (180 degrees Celsius).

In a large mixing bowl, whisk together milk and eggs. Combine the spinach, feta, and bread in a large mixing bowl. Gently toss until the milk mixture is absorbed by the bread. Fill a 13x9-inch glass or ceramic baking dish halfway with the mixture. Allow 20 to 30 minutes to cool at room temperature.

5. Bake for 35 minutes, or until set and lightly browned. Before serving, set aside for 5 to 10 minutes.

Breakfast Casserole with Tater Tots (n° 29)

20-Minute Preparation 1 hour and 10 minutes (total)

Number of servings: 10

• 12 ounces bulk turkey sausage • 12 cup chopped yellow onion • 1 cup chopped red bell pepper • 2 finely chopped garlic cloves • 8 large eggs • 12 cup whole milk • 2 teaspoons chili powder • 12 teaspoon cayenne pepper • 14 teaspoon ground pepper • 1 (28 ounce) package frozen potato tots

1 tablespoon chopped fresh chives • 34 cup shredded sharp Cheddar cheese

Directions

Preheat the oven to 350 degrees Fahrenheit (180 degrees Celsius). Using cooking spray, lightly coat a 9-by-13-inch baking dish. 2 teaspoons oil, heated over medium-high heat in a large nonstick skillet Cook, stirring and breaking up the meat with a wooden spoon, for 5 to 6 minutes, or until browned. Place on a plate lined with paper towels to absorb any excess liquid. Wipe the skillet clean with a paper towel but don't wash it.

2. Return the skillet to medium-high heat and add the remaining 1 teaspoon oil. Cook, stirring occasionally, for 7 minutes, or until onion and bell pepper are tender. Cook, stirring frequently, for 1 minute or until garlic is fragrant. In a separate bowl, combine the vegetables and the sausage that has been set aside.

3. In a large mixing bowl, mix together the eggs, milk, chili powder, cayenne, and pepper. Stir in the sausage-vegetable mixture. Fill the baking dish with the batter. Arrange potato tots in a single layer over the top. Add cheese on top.

4. Bake for 40 to 45 minutes, or until the cheese has browned and the casserole is set. Allow for a ten-minute resting period. Before serving, garnish with chives.

Prep Time: 45 minutes for 30. One-Pan Chicken Parmesan Pasta 45 minutes total Ingredients/Servings: 4

• 2 tablespoons extra-virgin olive oil, divided • 14 cup whole-wheat panko breadcrumbs • 1 tablespoon plus 1 teaspoon minced garlic, divided • 1 pound boneless, skinless chicken breast, cut into 1/2-inch pieces • 1 teaspoon Italian seasoning • 14 teaspoon salt • 3 cups low-sodium chicken broth • 11 12 cup crushed tomatoes • 8 ounces whole-wheat penne

Directions

1. In a large ovenproof skillet, heat 1 tablespoon oil on medium-high. 1 teaspoon garlic and 1 cup panko Cook, stirring constantly, for 1 to 2 minutes, or until the panko has turned golden brown. Set aside in a small mixing bowl. Remove the pan from the oven and wipe it down.

2. In a medium-high-heat pan, heat the remaining 1 tablespoon of oil. Add the remaining 1 tablespoon garlic, the chicken, Italian seasoning, and salt. Cook, stirring frequently, for 2 minutes, or until the outside of the chicken is no longer

pink. Combine the broth, tomatoes, and penne together in a large mixing bowl. Bring to a boil, then reduce to a low heat and cook, stirring occasionally, for 15 to 20 minutes, or until the penne is done and the sauce has thickened and reduced.

3. In the meantime, preheat the oven to 400°F and place an oven rack in the upper third. Raise the temperature of the broiler to high. Sprinkle mozzarella over the penne mixture once it's finished cooking. Place the pan under the broiler for about 1 minute, or until the mozzarella begins to bubble and brown. The panko mixture, Parmesan, and basil should be sprinkled on top.21. Cauliflower Rice and Spinach & Artichoke Casserole

20-Minute Preparation 45 minutes total Ingredients/Servings: 4

1 tablespoon extra-virgin olive oil • 1 pound boneless, skinless chicken breasts, cut into 1-inch pieces • 14 teaspoon salt • 14 teaspoon ground pepper • 2 garlic cloves, minced • 1 (14 ounce) can quartered artichoke hearts, drained and chopped • 12 cup unsalted chicken broth • 4 cups cauliflower rice • 3 cups coarsely chopped fresh spinach

• 1 cup part-skim mozzarella cheese, shredded

## Directions

Preheat the oven to 375 degrees Fahrenheit (190 degrees Celsius). Using cooking spray, lightly coat a 9-by-13-inch baking dish.

2. In a large pot, heat the oil on medium. Cook, stirring occasionally, until the chicken is opaque on all sides, about 4 minutes. Cook for 1 minute while stirring. Cook, stirring constantly, for 3 to 4 minutes, until the liquid has reduced and the chicken is cooked through. Remove the pan from the heat and stir in the cauliflower rice, spinach, yogurt, and 1/2 cup mozzarella cheese.

3. Spoon the remaining 1/2 cup mozzarella over the top of the mixture in the prepared baking dish. Cook for 20 to 25 minutes, or until the cheese is melted and browning in spots. Before serving, set aside for at least 5 minutes.

Preparation Time: 30 Minutes 22. Chicken and Zucchini Casserole 1 hour and 25 minutes total

Ingredients (servings): 8

• 3 tablespoons butter, divided • 2 pounds boneless, skinless chicken breast, cut into 1-inch pieces • 2 large zucchini, cut into 1/2-inch pieces • 1 large red bell pepper, chopped • 13 cup all-purpose flour • 1 cup no-salt-added chicken broth • 1 cup whole milk • 3 ounces reduced-fat cream cheese • 14 cups shredded part-skim mozzarella cheese, divided

Directions

Preheat the oven to 400 degrees Fahrenheit (200 degrees Celsius). In a large skillet on medium-high heat, melt 1 tablespoon butter. Cook, stirring occasionally, for about 8 minutes, until the chicken is well browned. In a medium bowl, place the chicken. Cook, stirring occasionally, until the zucchini and bell pepper begin to soften, about 4 minutes. In the same bowl as the chicken, add the zucchini mixture.

2. Remove the pan from the heat and add the remaining 2 tablespoons of butter. Cook, stirring constantly, for about 1 minute or until the flour begins to brown. Bring the broth and milk to a boil while constantly whisking. Remove from heat and stir in 3/4 cup mozzarella and cream cheese until thoroughly combined. Add the pepper and salt and stir to combine. Remove the liquid from the chicken and vegetable mixture and stir it into the cheese sauce. Fill a 2-quart baking dish halfway with water and set aside. Sprinkle the remaining 1/2 cup of cheese over the casserole and place it on a foil-lined baking sheet.

3. Bake for 20 to 25 minutes, or until top is browned and edges are bubbling. Before serving, set aside for 10 minutes.

Prep Time: 35 minutes for 23. Parmesan Mushroom Casserole 1 hour total Ingredients/Servings: 6

• 14 cup extra-virgin olive oil plus 1 tablespoon, divided • 1 cup chopped onion • 3 garlic cloves, minced • 2 pounds baby bella mushrooms, sliced • 3 tablespoons all-purpose flour • 34 teaspoon salt • 12 teaspoon ground pepper • 12 cup sour cream

Directions

Preheat the oven to 350 degrees Fahrenheit (180 degrees Celsius). Using cooking spray, spray an 8-inch-square baking dish.

2. In a large skillet, heat 1/4 cup oil on medium. Cook, stirring occasionally, for 3 minutes, or until onion is soft and beginning to brown. Cook for 1 minute while stirring. Add mushrooms in batches, stirring and cooking them down a little before adding another handful, until they've lost their opaqueness but there's still some liquid in the pan. Cook, stirring constantly, for 1 to 2 minutes, until the vegetables have thickened. Remove from the heat and stir in the sour

cream, 1/4 cup Parmesan cheese, 1/4 cup parsley, and the lemon juice. Place in the baking dish that has been prepared.

3. In a small mixing bowl, combine panko, the remaining 1 tablespoon oil, Parmesan, and parsley; toss to combine. Over the mushroom mixture, sprinkle the topping evenly. Cook for 20 to 25 minutes, or until the sauce has thickened and the breadcrumbs have lightly browned.

Dressing with lemon and scallions, no. 24

5 minutes to prepare 5 minutes in total Ingredients/Servings: 6

• 6 tbsp extra-virgin olive oil • 3 tbsp lemon juice • 2 tbsp chopped shallot • 1 tbsp honey • 12 tbsp salt • 14 tbsp ground pepper

1. In a small mixing bowl, combine the olive oil, lemon juice, shallot, honey, salt, and pepper.

25. Parmesan-Crusted Lentil and Vegetable Soup

15-Minute Preparation 40 minutes total Ingredients/Servings: 6

• 2 tablespoons extra-virgin olive oil • 3 cups fresh or frozen chopped onion, carrot, and celery mix • 4 garlic cloves, chopped • 4 cups low-sodium vegetable or chicken broth • 12 cup green or brown lentils • 1 (15-ounce) can unsalted diced tomatoes, undrained • 2 teaspoons finely chopped fresh thyme • 12 teaspoon salt • 12 teaspoon ground pepper • 12 teaspoon crushed red pepper

• Chopped fresh flat-leaf parsley for garnish • 12 tablespoons red-wine vinegar Directions

2. In a Dutch oven or a large pot, heat the oil on medium. Cook, stirring occasionally, for 6 to 10 minutes, until onion, carrot, and celery mixture is softened. Cook, stirring frequently, for 30 seconds, until garlic is fragrant.

3. Add the broth, lentils, tomatoes, thyme, salt, pepper, crushed red pepper, and, if using, Parmesan rind. On medium-high heat, bring to a boil. Reduce to medium-low heat; cover and cook, stirring occasionally, for 15 to 25 minutes, or until lentils are almost tender, adding water as needed to thin to desired consistency.

4. Add kale to the mix. Cook for 5 to 10 minutes, covered, until kale is tender. If you're using Parmesan rind, remove it

and throw it away. Vinegar should be added now. Split the money in half.

Mediterranean Diet in a Slow Cooker (#26) 15-Minute Stew Prep

6 hours and 45 minutes total

Ingredients/Servings: 6

• 2 (14 ounce) cans no-salt-added fire-roasted diced tomatoes • 3 cups low-sodium vegetable broth • 1 cup coarsely chopped onion • 34 cup chopped carrot • 4 garlic cloves, minced • 1 teaspoon dried oregano • 34 teaspoon salt • 12 teaspoon crushed red pepper • 14 teaspoon ground pepper • 1 (15 ounce) can no-salt-added chickpeas, rinsed, divided

• 3 tbsp extra-virgin olive oil • 6 lemon wedges • 3 tbsp extra-virgin olive oil (Optional) Directions

In a 4-quart slow cooker, mix together the tomatoes, broth, onion, carrot, garlic, oregano, salt, crushed red pepper, and pepper. Cook for 6 hours on low, covered.

2. In a small bowl, pour 1/4 cup of the slow cooker's cooking liquid. 2 tablespoons chickpeas, mashed until smooth with a

fork

3. Toss the remaining whole chickpeas into the slow cooker with the mashed chickpeas, kale, and lemon juice. To combine everything, whisk it together. Cook, covered, on Low for about 30 minutes, or until the kale is tender.

4. Divide the stew among 6 bowls and drizzle with olive oil. Basil leaves can be added as a finishing touch. If you'd like, garnish with lemon wedges.

Chhole is number 27. (Chickpea Curry)

15 minutes total Ingredients/Servings: 6

• 6 tablespoons canola oil or grapeseed oil • 2 teaspoons ground coriander • 2 teaspoons ground cumin • 12 teaspoon ground turmeric • 2 14 cups no-salt-added canned diced tomatoes with their juice (from a 28-ounce can) • 34 teaspoon kosher salt • 2 15-ounce cans chickpeas, rinsed

• For garnish, fresh cilantro

Directions

1. In a food processor, finely mince the serrano, garlic, and ginger. Re-pulse after scraping down the sides. Pulse the onion until it's finely chopped but not watery.

2. In a large saucepan, heat the oil on medium-high. Cook, stirring occasionally, for 3 to 5 minutes, or until the onion mixture has softened. Cook, stirring constantly, for 2 minutes with coriander, cumin, and turmeric.

3. Pulse the tomatoes until they are finely chopped in a food processor. Salt and add to the pan. Cook, stirring occasionally, for 4 minutes at a low simmer. Reduce heat to a low heat, add the chickpeas and garam masala, cover, and cook for 5 minutes more, stirring occasionally. If desired, garnish with chopped cilantro.

28. Casserole de Petits Fours de Noel de Noel de Noel

20-Minute Preparation 1 hour and 10 minutes (total)

Ingredients (servings): 8

• 14 cup chopped sun-dried tomatoes • 1 tablespoon extra-virgin olive oil • 2 garlic cloves, finely chopped • 12 teaspoon crushed red pepper • 1 teaspoon lemon zest • 2 cups low-fat milk • 5 large eggs • 1 cup crumbled feta cheese • 12 ounces rustic whole-wheat bread, torn into 1-inch pieces (about 8 cups)

## Directions

1. Place the spinach in a clean kitchen towel and wring out as much liquid as possible over the sink. In a medium mixing bowl, combine the spinach and artichoke hearts.

2. In a small skillet over low heat, cook the tomatoes, oil, garlic, crushed red pepper, and lemon zest, stirring frequently, until fragrant and golden brown, 3 to 4 minutes. Add the spinach mixture to it and mix well.

3. Preheat the oven to 350 degrees Fahrenheit (180 degrees Celsius).

In a large mixing bowl, whisk together milk and eggs. Combine the spinach, feta, and bread in a large mixing bowl. Gently toss until the milk mixture is absorbed by the bread. Fill a 13x9-inch glass or ceramic baking dish halfway with the mixture. Allow 20 to 30 minutes to cool at room temperature.

5. Bake for 35 minutes, or until set and lightly browned. Before serving, set aside for 5 to 10 minutes.

Breakfast Casserole with Tater Tots (n° 29)

20-Minute Preparation 1 hour and 10 minutes (total)

Number of servings: 10

• 12 ounces bulk turkey sausage • 12 cup chopped yellow onion • 1 cup chopped red bell pepper • 2 finely chopped garlic cloves • 8 large eggs • 12 cup whole milk • 2 teaspoons chili powder • 12 teaspoon cayenne pepper • 14 teaspoon ground pepper • 1 (28 ounce) package frozen potato tots

1 tablespoon chopped fresh chives • 34 cup shredded sharp Cheddar cheese

Directions

Preheat the oven to 350 degrees Fahrenheit (180 degrees Celsius). Using cooking spray, lightly coat a 9-by-13-inch baking dish. 2 teaspoons oil, heated over medium-high heat in a large nonstick skillet Cook, stirring and breaking up the meat with a wooden spoon, for 5 to 6 minutes, or until browned. Place on a plate lined with paper towels to absorb any excess liquid. Wipe the skillet clean with a paper towel but don't wash it.

2. Return the skillet to medium-high heat and add the remaining 1 teaspoon oil. Cook, stirring occasionally, for 7 minutes, or until onion and bell pepper are tender. Cook, stirring frequently, for 1 minute or until garlic is fragrant. In a separate bowl, combine the vegetables and the sausage that has been set aside.

3. In a large mixing bowl, mix together the eggs, milk, chili powder, cayenne, and pepper. Stir in the sausage-vegetable mixture. Fill the baking dish with the batter. Arrange potato tots in a single layer over the top. Add cheese on top.

4. Bake for 40 to 45 minutes, or until the cheese has browned and the casserole is set. Allow for a ten-minute resting period. Before serving, garnish with chives.

Prep Time: 45 minutes for 30. One-Pan Chicken Parmesan Pasta 45 minutes total Ingredients/Servings: 4

• 2 tablespoons extra-virgin olive oil, divided • 14 cup whole-wheat panko breadcrumbs • 1 tablespoon plus 1 teaspoon minced garlic, divided • 1 pound boneless, skinless chicken breast, cut into 1/2-inch pieces • 1 teaspoon Italian seasoning • 14 teaspoon salt • 3 cups low-sodium chicken broth • 11 12 cup crushed tomatoes • 8 ounces whole-wheat penne

## Directions

1. In a large ovenproof skillet, heat 1 tablespoon oil on medium-high. 1 teaspoon garlic and 1 cup panko Cook, stirring constantly, for 1 to 2 minutes, or until the panko has turned golden brown. Set aside in a small mixing bowl. Remove the pan from the oven and wipe it down.

2. In a medium-high-heat pan, heat the remaining 1 tablespoon of oil. Add the remaining 1 tablespoon garlic, the chicken, Italian seasoning, and salt. Cook, stirring frequently, for 2 minutes, or until the outside of the chicken is no longer pink. Combine the broth, tomatoes, and penne together in a large mixing bowl. Bring to a boil, then reduce to a low heat and cook, stirring occasionally, for 15 to 20 minutes, or until the penne is done and the sauce has thickened and reduced.

3. In the meantime, preheat the oven to 400°F and place an oven rack in the upper third. Raise the temperature of the broiler to high. Sprinkle mozzarella over the penne mixture once it's finished cooking. Place the pan under the broiler for about 1 minute, or until the mozzarella begins to bubble and brown. The panko mixture, Parmesan, and basil should be sprinkled on top.

CPSIA information can be obtained
at www.ICGtesting.com
Printed in the USA
LVHW020741160322
713569LV00008B/929